Therapeutic And Beauty

Staples From Home

VEVINE GOLDSON

DEDICATION

This book is dedicated to my fans and friends. You have been such an amazing inspiration! You know who you are.

So here is a handy compilation with some of my favourite topics to stash on your book shelves.

Table of Contents

Castor oil

Everybody likes a bit of indulgence and looking our fantastic best, but when you have not much time left to visit the beauty parlour, you have to just DIY. So here I have compiled for you some quick to whip up alternatives. I have been using black castor oil for many years and have not been disappointed. This oil is notorious for its many benefits, and has been passed down from many generations and folk healers. The history of castor oil dates way back to Africa when the ancient Pharaonic times the brown and black Egyptians used it as a natural remedy; In the fourth century B.C. the Egyptians and the Kushites "roasted them and then boil them down and collected the oil.

The benefits are endless. Castor oil is antifungal and antibacterial; the oil has many skin healing properties and can be used as an anti-bacterial remedy when applied to affected areas.. As a beauty treatment when it is used topically, it can slow down the process of aging and make spots less visible. It penetrates the skin intensely and stimulates the production of collagen and elastin.

When ingested It is also known to stir bowel movement so pregnant mothers should avoid taking it and people that are on medication should consult their doctors first before ingestion. Growing up and While spending time with elder relatives, I remember them giving me castor oil to boost my immune system, lower bowel movements and also as a topical treatment for inflamed skin to speed up healing and as a disinfectant for bruises and cuts. After eating all that Christmas treats I was given spoon full of castor oil to purge the blood and balance the digestive system.

Castor oil is also an exceptional remedy for stimulating hair growth. Massaging your scalp with it can give you thicker and longer hair. The oil increases circulation to the follicles, leading to stronger and faster hair growth. Castor-oil has omega-9 essential fatty acids that promotes shiny healthy hair. It also helps reduce split ends, controls hair breakage, and conditions and moisturizes your hair.

The castor oil purifies the skin and helps to get rid of parasites and toxins that can sometimes stunt hair growth. It also helps to repair extremely damaged hair and smooth out split ends. It is used as a hot oil treatment. Warm enough oil in a microwave pour and rub thoroughly through hair and scalp, then place a steaming cap on the head. Leave on for fifteen to thirty minutes, then shampoo condition and style hair as usual.

Apart from making all those Christmas puddings fry festivals and journey cakes with cornmeal, it can also be used topically as a beauty treatment. Cornmeal when mixed with other ingredients from your kitchen is considered an excellent exfoliator and skin smoother and is a very inexpensive way to treat your skin.

Why this is good for skin?

Corn and cornmeal contain zinc, manganese, iron, copper, magnesium, and cornmeal contains trace minerals just like selenium.

Honey is naturally antibacterial liquid, so it's great for acne treatment and the prevention of aging . It is also Full of antioxidants, which makes it great for slowing down aging, giving your skin a more youthful glow.

Eggs are loaded with high-quality proteins, vitamins, minerals, good fats and various traces of other nutrients.

Cornmeal eggs and honey: I first was introduced to this treatment at the age of eighteen when I was attending modelling classes. I was spending a lot of time in the sun and my skin became irritated and dry. My mentor was the first person that noticed the dryness in my skin and he told me about the cornmeal eggs and honey treatment, and I have never looked back. This not only heals the skin of dryness but gets rid of excess oil, works as an excellent moisturizer and evens out your skin.

Cornmeal scrub has always be good for a long time but be careful not to mistake cornmeal with corn starch, you will notice that cornmeal is yellow in colour and corn-starch is white.

Mix half a cup of cornmeal two large spoons full of honey and the white of an egg into a paste. Before using your scrub makes sure your skin is bare and clean first before application. Wash face to remove old makeup and dirt then apply your cornmeal scrub.

You can leave it on for as long as you want but I keep mine on for thirty minutes. After wash you will notice that your skin is feeling smooth and silky. It gets rid of excess oil and it does not dry out your skin. It can be used on the face and any other parts of the body. Apply on and scrub face but do not scrub too hard, and let it stay for desired minutes then wash face and pat dry. You will see and feel the difference on your skin!

Sugar scrub mixed with extra virgin olive oil: Sugar is one of the most natural staple in our kitchen, and is one of the easiest to work with, and it is also natural source of glycolic acid. Over the years there has been numerous researches, and it has shown that sugar contains glycolic acid which is used to treat sun-damaged and aging skin. It eliminates the roughness in extremely dry skin especial elbows and heels. Sugar pulls moisture into the skin which deeply penetrates the epidermis. It hydrates the skin thus helping to keep moisture in.

Extra Virgin Olive Oil is The Healthiest Fat, and super healthy, and is widely used around the world. Not only is it good for you internally but Olive oil is considered a liquid gold and has been used to treat the skin since back in the time of Cleopatra, Olive oil contains three major antioxidants: vitamin E, polyphenols, and Phytosterols. It is said to lower your blood pressure, and reduces inflammation and may help prevent unwanted blood clotting.

For people at risk of heart disease olive oil is most definitely one of the most healthy food to consume, but make sure that it is the real deal, extra virgin olive oil and not a diluted version that is mixed with other oils. Researches have shown that olive oil can help to fight cancer and Alzheimer's disease.

It is full of antioxidants and that makes it good for your nails skin and hair. People that lives in Mediterranean countries have a fairly low risk of cancer and some have speculated that olive oil has something to do with that low volume of cancer rate.

When anti-oxidants is applied to the skin it helps to slow down premature aging. It fights the appearance of aging and leaves skin with a natural healthy texture and glow. The vitamin E in the oil helps to restore the skins elasticity and soothes, softens and protects it from ultraviolet rays. It removes dead skin cells leaving the skin to glow naturally, and is used for cuticle and nail care.

If you have extremely sensitive skin you can opt for Brown sugar which is softer than granulated. Wash your face and make sure your makeup is completely removed before applying the scrub. Lots of women use it to remove dirt and makeup. Sugar Scrub Ingredients

1/2 cup sugar (white or brown sugar)

1/2 cup oil (olive oil) stir and mix well then store in a jar. Use whenever you feel the need for a facial.

The cucumber: Cucumber is known to be a vegetable but it is actually a nutritious fruit and there are many ways you can enjoy cucumbers, but First and foremost here is why Staying up late and not getting a good night's sleep, smoking, drinking and hard partying are responsible for people having bags under their eyes" and This long edible fresh tasting fruit is not only good for consumption but there are benefits to using it on the skin.

It is widely used around the world and in beauty salons as a treatment that can reduce the effects of swelling and puffiness around the eyes.

Cucumbers are low in calories, have 95% water, and have fibre, as well as vitamins and minerals contain antioxidants, including flavonoids and tannins, so in essence it is a great moisturizer for the skin. Cucumber has natural firming ingredients and many cosmetic and skin care products have cucumber in it.

Here are some of the top health benefits that cucumber is known to have.

1. Eating cucumbers may lead to many potential health benefits, including weight loss, balanced hydration, digestive regularity and lower blood sugar levels.
2. Cucumber helps to Protect your brain from neurological diseases
3. Fight inflammation in the body and reduce the risk of cancer.
4. Cucumbers are rich in water, and their skin contains insoluble fibre. Both water and fibre help food to move through the digestive tract quicker and more easily, helping prevent constipation.
5. Has vitamin k is essential for bone health, as low vitamin K intakes have been associated with a higher risk for bone fracture.

If you are suffering from redness and irritation, Cut two slices of cucumber and place on each eyes. You can also soak cotton balls in cucumber juice and apply to the eyes. Grated cucumbers can be used as a remedy to treat freckles tighten open pores cleanse and tones the skin.

Do not forget to have a tall glass of cucumber juice because Cucumber juice is enriched with magnesium, fibre, and potassium, and have been known to control the effects of blood pressure. So if you are troubled with low blood pressure or high blood pressure, cucumber juice can effectively regulate both of the conditions in a natural way.

Apart from being healthy oil for cooking, coconut oil has many other benefits. Coconut oil is rich in saturated fats which got a bad rap a few decades ago but as time goes by new researches has shown that it was refined coconut oil that contained these bad fats, and the unrefined organic virgin coconut oil is the healthiest choice.

The saturated fats present in coconut oil have antimicrobial properties which in turn help to fight various bacteria, fungi, and parasites that can cause indigestion. It is good for the digestive system and help to prevent indigestion including irritable bowel syndrome.

The benefits of this oil when used on the skin:

The best coconut oil to use is extra virgin coconut oil raw and organic. Coconut oil has anti-aging properties and is widely used as an important ingredient in several skin care creams because when the oil is applied topically to the skin, it moisturizes repairs the skin and helps to protect against sun damage.

Coconut oil does not clog the pores and can be used as an exfoliator, when it is used together with grainy agents it DE- clogs and removes dead skin cells from the surface without drying out your skin. Your skin will be soft smooth and a more evened out skin tone, while improving the texture of the skin.

Coconut oil contains anti-bacterial and anti-fungal properties, which not only protects against dandruff and lice, but also cleanses the scalp and hair follicles.

Coconut oil is said to rapidly grow hair thicker longer faster, vitamins and essential fatty acids naturally found in coconut oil nourishes the scalp while stimulating new hair growth. Using coconut oil regularly will over time leave your hair thicker, luscious, shiny and soft, while protecting it from heat and environmental damage.

To deep condition your hair pour enough amount that suits the length of your hair into a container, then try heating the oil in the microwave rub through hair massaging and smoothing it out from scalp to strand, then place a plastic cap on. You can leave it one for thirty to sixty minutes or if you wish overnight for deep intense conditioning.

Lemons are considered a super-food but that is an understatement, lemons are extremely good for your intestine and outer intestine for a variety of reasons. While lemons are known for their acidic taste, they're remarkably a good source of an alkaline food that can help balance your body's ph. Lemons have anti-oxidants in the juice and skin which is used to treat conditions that can sometimes result in severe ailments.

The flavonoids in the lemon are an antiseptic that is used to treat bacterial infections and several other different disorders. The pulp from the lemon and the skin contains pectin that is used to help with high cholesterol levels and low sugar levels in people that suffer from diabetes. When the pectin goes through alteration it can help to treat the spread of certain types of cancer.

Lemons are Rich in Bioflavonoids which can be found in some vegetables and fruits and they are also an excellent source of vitamin B6, iron and potassium, folic acid, phosphorus, calcium, copper, magnesium, manganese, zinc, fibre and vitamin c.

Here are some good things about lemons to note.

The juice has antibacterial agents.

Adding lemons to your meal can make it healthier and tastier.

The bioflavonoids in lemon protect against damage caused by free radicals, and enhance the antioxidant effects of some nutrients.

The flavonoids can help protect against heart disease. maintain capillaries and help the blood clot.

For mouth ulcers gaggle with warm water lemon and a bit of salt.

Rubbing lemon on affected areas of acne skin can help to lighten aged spots and even out skin tone. Although it dries out pimples, those with sensitive skin need to be careful when using this treatment. In the summer we tend to eat a lot of sweet treats including ice cream, cakes, and sweet fruits which tend to attract a lot of fruit flies. When that occur you can squeeze a few lemons in a jar add some warm water then pour the contents in a spray bottle. Shake well and spray the areas that are attracting the flies.

Some cuisines are just not as tasty without mayonnaise, What would our burgers, sandwiches and coleslaws taste like without this creamy and very popular dressing ? But is this creamy condiment healthy for you? According to the American Egg Board, approximately 8 billion eggs are used in the USA to make commercial mayonnaise. Mayonnaise is usually made by whipping together eggs, oil, and vinegar, so it rapidly increases the calorie count of anything it's used in. But it's so mouth-watering and delicious!

One tablespoon of traditional mayonnaise contains about 90 calories and 90 milligrams of sodium, and if consumed on a daily basis it may lead to weight gain and obesity, and excess cholesterol intake can lead to build-ups in your arteries. But do not panic my dear mayonnaise lovers because not all mayonnaise are made with high calorie ingredients, Just for peace of mind, egg-free mayonnaise is also available for vegans and vegetarians. It is made with soy milk, starch, and a few other low fat ingredients. Although it is lighter, it tastes just as good.

The egg yolks are usually replaced with ingredients like soy milk or starch which is lower in fat. Yes there is a lot of fat in traditional mayonnaise but that doesn't mean it is all bad, Some mayonnaise are made with egg white, while most are made with the whole egg – yolk and white, low fat mayo is a much healthier choice.

But apart from all that is delectable about mayonnaise, there are so many other uses that this food condiment can be used for. Did you know that mayonnaise can be used to treat damaged hair? Yes mayonnaise is good for hair use. Here is why. Mayonnaise is packed with ingredients that help to nourish your hair, The proteins in the eggs nourishes the strands and promote healthy hair growth.

Mayonnaise also kills hair lice, when Evenly spread on your hair and scalp.

Mayonnaise-And-Olive-Oil-Hair-treatment. Whip up 1/2 cup virgin Olive Oil and 1/2 cup Mayonnaise, apply to hair cover with a steaming cap and leave on for thirty minutes.

Mayonnaise-And-egg--Hair-treatment. Whip 2 to 3 eggs, and half cup mayonnaise, coat hair root right to the tips leave for thirty minutes, rinse then rinse.

Bananas is said to be one of the most popular fruit in the UK. On average most UK residents eat 10kg of bananas each year (about 100 bananas). The most popular type of banana is the long slim, yellow skinned variety of sweet bananas, and the larger ones which are called plantains are boiled and cut into thin slices and fried to make plantain chips. Bananas are also used in the same way to make chips known as banana chips.

Bananas are power packed with potassium, vitamin B6, vitamin C, fibre and carbohydrate. Ripe bananas are said to have a lower water content than most fruit, typically they have more calories as well as a higher sugar content compared to other fruits that are not from the tropics. When bananas are not ripe they have a higher starch content, and when they become ripe, the starch is converted to sugar that gives the fruit its sweet taste.

Bananas are grown in hot climates, so it is difficult for the plant to survive in the cold, so If they are kept in the fridge, the enzymes that causes them to ripen are neutralized, and The skin might eventually become blackened, but if you prefer an un-ripe banana you might want to keep them in the fridge. Bananas and plantains are picked green and transported from the tropics and set to store and ripen at room temperature, or when placed inside plastic bags.

Bananas can have great benefits for your hair and skin. Bananas can tighten open pores, shrink acne and the potassium in bananas leave your skin well hydrated. When used in hair the minerals and vitamins in its contents balances the PH of the scalp and hair.

The banana hair mask: Here is how to make it.

Get one to two bananas and some virgin olive oil, how much bananas and oil you use will depend on how thick or long your hair is. Peel the bananas and placed in a bowl, add one large spoon full of olive oil. Whip or blend it together into a smooth liquid, make sure there are no lumps. Apply to the hair and scalp, let it stay for 15 to 20 minutes then rinse.

Here is how to make a banana face mask:

Get one ripe banana and 1 ½ to two teaspoons raw honey. Squash the banana and honey until they are equally blend, apply to clean face. Let it stay for 10 to 20 minutes then wash off, pat face dry. Your skin will look soft and moisture.

Tea is an ancient beverage and there is a wide variety of tea to suit every palate. Tea is a very versatile drink and is the second most widely consumed beverage in the world after water. Tea isn't just a calming and enjoyable hot and cold beverage, but it is also known to have extra-ordinary therapeutic properties, and is sometimes seen as a super drink that is better than drinking pure clear water.

Our ancestors have been drinking tea for ages and have been using tea herbs to cure illnesses and to soothe aches and pains. Researches have shown that consuming certain types of teas especially green tea can help to fight diseases and lengthen life.

Tea is power packed with high concentration of antioxidants the most dominant one is called polyphenols, which may contribute to the prevention of cancer, osteoporosis, and cardiovascular diseases. A study that was carried out in Japan a country where green tea is popular and widely consumed found drinking green tea substantially lowered the risk of perishing from cardiovascular disease. 3o% lower risk in women, and 23% lower risk in men.

Green tea is also said to boost brain power and help with deeper concentration, so people that are studying should stock up on green tea. It can also help to relax the muscles and heal people that suffer from anxieties and constant fatigue. Because of its L-thianine which is an amino acid that occurs naturally in the plant, that helps to boost alpha wave in the brains that leads to discreet awareness.

People that are troubled with athlete foot can use tea as an effective cure.

Here is how to use tea for athlete foot. Put a few tea bags in a pan with water and brew it strongly then pour the contents into a foot pan and when the tea is warm enough place foot into the bath pan and soak. Do this daily until the athlete's foot is cured.

If you have not been sleeping well or have been partying hard and developed tired and puffy eyes, here is how to revitalize them.

Soak two four tea bags in warm water and place them over your eyes, make sure to close your eyes first, let the bags stay on your closed eyes for 15 to 30 minutes. The tannins in the tea bags help to decrease puffiness and calm and soothe tired eyes.

Develop an unsightly boil? Here is what to do. Place a wet tea bag over the affected area, let it stay overnight, and the boil will burst and begin to drain by itself. You can use a warm tea bag for this purpose.

Baking Soda is a crystalline salt and the salt has been known by many other names such as baking soda, bread soda, cooking soda, and bicarbonate of soda. It has long been known as a raising agent and is popularly used in foods. For decades baking soda has been used as a rising agent when baking bread and pastry. This powdery agent (sodium bicarbonate) when mixed with acid makes bubbles and gives off a carbon dioxide gas which makes the dough and pastry rise.

Baking soda is known as anchorite, that is known as a form of natural mineral matron. Natrona encompasses large amounts of sodium bicarbonate and has been used subsequently since the days of prehistoric times as a cleansing agent which also deodorizes and soothes. Yes baking soda is amazingly good for your health and home too!

There are many health benefits associated with using baking soda. It can be used to ease tiredness in the feet, it can be used to remove dead skin cells from the face and other areas of the skin and can be used to remove splinter and also illuminate Odours From Vacuum Cleaners, cars and and around the home.

You can eliminate these odours from vehicles by sprinkling baking soda directly on fabric the seats and carpets. Wait 20 to 30 minutes before hovering up the baking soda from the vehicles; if the odour is strong you can leave it overnight before vacuuming. This can also be used to deodorize pet beddings cat litter and dog kennels. Sprinkle on beddings and pet areas, let stand for some minutes depends on how strong the odour is then remove the baking soda.

To clean the skin on some vegetables and fruits, you can sprinkle a little baking soda on a damp flannel, sponge or soft cloth and scrub gently.

This very popular household staple can also be used as an alternative to spa treatments.

As a hair treatment here is what to do.

Sprinkle one quart amount of baking soda into a bulk of your favourite shampoo. When you wash and rinse your hair you will notice that it is more manageable shinier and healthy.

As a skin treatment here is what to do. Pour three parts baking soda into water, then mix into a paste. Apply unto your face and gently scrub in circular motion, then rinse with warm water. You can do the same for unsightly tan marks.

Vinegar is an acidic clear liquid made and used by people throughout history and has been produced through fermentation. It has a sour taste and Traces of it have been found in Egyptian urns from around 3000 BC. There are different kinds of vinegar out there a variety includes Chinese black vinegar, a lighter version of black vinegar made from rice is produced in Japan, coconut vinegar, sugar cane vinegar, balsamic vinegar, apple cider vinegar, fruit vinegar most of which are produced in Europe, persimmon vinegar from Korea and the list goes on.

Folklore has it that during the black plague that occurred in France; a group of four thieves were able to rob infected people without catching the infection. Their secret was revealed to a judge when asked, they told that a medicine woman sold them a portion of vinegar that was brewed in garlic and sour red wine today known as vinegar.

Commercial vinegar that are distributed you will find most do not exceed 5% if the vinegar is over that percentage careful handling is needed as it can damage skin tissues if not handled with care. Vinegar has been known to be beneficial in a number of ways, and In Canada the maximum acid of vinegars must be between 4.1% and 12.3%. It has a great variety of uses industrial, culinary, medical, and domestic uses.

Vinegar is frequently used in food provision; it is commonly used in the making of pickles, chutney and salad dressings. It is one of the main ingredients in sauces such as mustard, ketchup, and also mayonnaise and is very popular in Britain as a condiment for fish and chips. Drinks are also made using vinegar one popular among the Greeks is known as oxymel a traditional Persian juice.

Vinegar has been reputed to have strong antibacterial properties. Researches have shown that 5% vinegar kills bacteria and moulds, it is 90% effectively good at reducing mould and 99.9% effective against bacteria, it also kills bacteria and moulds on produce when applied to affected areas.

To remove stubborn stains on carpets. Mix half cup of white vinegar and three table spoons of salt apply when dry hoover the spot.

Clean kettle with by adding three cups of white vinegar let boil and sit overnight, then rinse thoroughly before use.

For those that are troubled with dandruff Mix together half cup apple cider vinegar and equal water. Massage into your scalp shampoo and rinse.

Melons is said to be originated from Africa and the south of Asia, and One of the first fruit to be made popular from early ancient times. The seeds are said to appear in the bronze age in 1350 and 1120 BC but during travelling and trade they started to appear in Europe during the Roman Empire era. It is also a low calorie fruit that is high in nutrients, which includes carotenoids, vitamin C and A. The minerals and vitamins can benefit your heart and brain health.

There are a variety of melons. Japanese melons, including the Sprite melon, Korean melon, a yellow melon with white lines, Tiger melon, yellow and black striped melon from Turkey Sharlyn melons, summer melons, winter melons and the list goes on with different cross breeds of the fruit from Mexico etc.

Melon gradually began to appear in Europe toward the end of the Roman Empire. However recent discoveries of melon seeds dated between 1350 and 1120 BC in Neuralgic sacred wells have shown that melons were first brought to Europe by the neuralgic civilization of Sardinia during the Bronze Age.

 Melons were among the earliest plants to be domesticated in both the Old and New Worlds. Early European settlers in the New World are recorded as growing honeydew and casaba melons as early as the 1600s.

Melon has a lot of beneficial nutrients in its contents that can rejuvenate and revitalize hair and skin. The A and C vitamins in the melon is beneficial for skin and hair.

If your skin appears to be tired and dry you can boost moisture, by dampening a cotton bud in the juices of melon and apply to clean face. Remember to wash your face before apply the melon juices. You will begin to appear smoother and hydrated.

According to health news, the high content of carotenoids in melon fruit can prevent cancer and lower the risk of lung cancer. Drinking melon punch and juices will be beneficial for your health as researches has shown that it can prevent the growth of certain types of cancer by killing the cells, so try to get more melon in your system by adding more of it to your diet.

Melons can also cure kidney disease according to researches diuretic properties of melon are beneficial in curing kidney disease and are very good for your digestive system. Watermelon contains both Fibre and water contents that is good for digestion.

Avocado

13

Avocados are grown in warm climate like the tropics and Mediterranean throughout the world and are also known as pear especially in the Caribbean islands like Jamaica and Barbados. The tree has a long history of farming in Central and South America, possibly beginning as early as 5,000 BC. There are variations of avocado that are different in colour, shape, and size. Avocados contains a lot of fibre, vitamins and minerals such as vitamin K, vitamin E, vitamin C and B-vitamins, potassium, and copper, that is good for eye and age related diseases and is a great choice for pregnant women.

Most are pear shaped with green smooth skin and fleshy green pulp but there is a smaller variety known as criollo the native undomesticated variety of avocado which is very small with gritty black skin and contains a large seed. The similarity with banana, avocado is a climacteric fruit, which matures on the tree, but ripens off the tree.

In the United Kingdom, the avocado became available during the 1960s when introduced by Sainsbury's under the name 'avocado pear'.

Mexico was the world's largest avocado growing country, producing several times more than the second largest producer but Peru has now become the largest supplier of avocados imported to the European Union.

Avocados are often use in flavoursome exotic dishes in some cultures, and are a relative novelty in Portuguese-speaking countries, such as Brazil, where the traditional preparation is mashed with sugar and lime, and eaten as a dessert or snack.

Due to its effective nutrients, it is helpful for those seeking to lose weight. Eating avocados can also reduce the risk of cardiovascular disease.

Avocado exfoliator how to.

Mix half avocado with a ripe banana and an egg yolk into a smooth paste. Apply to face for thirty minutes rinse off and pat skin dry. Many beauty enthusiasts have attributed their improved skin condition to the use of avocado facial masks.

Avocado hair mask how to.

Mix avocado, extra virgin oil and honey. Whip until smooth apply to hair cover with cap for thirty minutes, then rinse.

The orange is a sweet and juicy pulpy fruit that is loaded with vitamin c and other nutrients. The strong antioxidant found in oranges can also help to combat the formation of free radicals known to cause cancer. The fibre, potassium, vitamin C and choline content in oranges all support heart health. The antioxidant vitamin C, that is found in orange when it is applied directly to the skin, can help to fight sun damaged skin and reduce wrinkles and improve the skins elasticity, because it plays a vital role in collagen formation.

Due to unhealthy lifestyles and the consumption of junk foods the arteries become blocked, which can lead to heart attack and cardiovascular diseases. The flavonoids in oranges reduce cholesterol and prevent your arteries from getting blocked.

Researches have shown that the nutrients help to keep the immune system healthy and shorten certain types of illnesses. Eating one orange a day can reduce the risk of mouth, larynx and stomach cancers by up to 50 per- cent, according to research by the Commonwealth Scientific and Industrial Research Organization.

Scientific evidence has shown that organically grown oranges have up to 30 per- cent more vitamin C even when the organic oranges were smaller and the ripened oranges may have a higher antioxidant substance than their unripe fruit.

The orange peel has antibacterial agents that are great for treating acne prone and oily skin. When use regularly It lightens stubborn discolorations, and leave the skin with a nice even tone and texture.

For discolorations and pigmentation here is what to do.

As we age, our skin suffers from free radical damage. Oranges are power packed with antioxidants and Vitamin C that stimulate collagen which leaves you with fresh clear looking younger skin.

Add 2 table spoons of orange peel powder and a few drops of lime and two table spoons of honey. Mix them together into a smooth paste then apply to face and rub in circular motion. Let it stay on the skin for 15 to 20 minutes then rinse with warm water. Pat face dry.

If you suffer from dandruff here is what to do

Orange peel can reduce dandruff. Make a paste of orange peel and lemon and apply on the scalp and hair for 15 to 20 minutes before shampooing. Shampoo Condition then rinse.

Oats: oatmeal is one of the best condiment in our kitchen, it is considered one of the best heart food thanks to its levels of beta-glucan, Oats provide important minerals. Nutrient-rich oatmeal contains thiamine, magnesium, phosphorus, zinc, manganese, selenium, and iron. It is great for those looking to lose a few pounds . "If you're eating oatmeal to lower your cholesterol, you'll want to eat about a cup-and-a-half a day.

Oatmeal Face Mask.

This treatment is especially good for the skin because the honey and lemon hydrates the skin while the oats remove dead skin cells and the vinegar regulate the PH balance.

Add three table spoons of oatmeal two table spoon of honey one table spoon of vinegar and quarter cup of warm water. Mix together into a paste then apply to clean face.

Colloidal oatmeal (3 tablespoons) rinse 20 minutes time with warm water.

Oatmeal body scrub how to.

Add quarter cup oatmeal, one large spoon of honey and some goats milk. Squash and mix together. When it's time for bath or shower you can use it as a body scrub. Avoid scrubbing soft fleshy skin to much. You may scrub as long as you want until you are satisfied. I keep the left overs refrigerated in a glass jar with lid make sure to use it up within one week.

Oatmeal foot spa.

Add half cup of fresh milk and one cup of oats in a foot tub.

Two spoons full of honey.

Throw in a few smooth pebbles

and rose petals of your choice. When you are done you can use a pumice stone to remove the rest of dead skin from underneath your foot bottom.

Enjoy nice smooth soft feet!

Simple oatmeal facial scrub

Mix oatmeal into a paste with milk of your choice. Apply to clean face, let it stay for 15 to 20 minutes. Rinse face with warm water and pat dry with a towel. Oatmeal helps to remove redness while it softens the skin.

Turmeric grows wild in the forests of South and Southeast Asia where it is collected for use in traditional medicine; and is widely used as a key ingredient in Asian cuisine. Turmeric is used mostly in savoury dishes, but is also used in some sweet dishes, such as the cake and other pastries. A perennial herbaceous plant that can grow up to three feet tall. The branches range from yellow to orange. In China the flowering time is usually in August. The long inflorescence stem contains many flowers. The bracts are light green and ovate to oblong with a blunt upper end with a length of 3 to 5 cm.

Turmeric is used in traditional recipes as an agent to impart a golden yellow colour and flavour. The leaves of the plant are sometimes used to wrap and cook food which adds a distinctive essence. The leaves are mainly used in this way in areas where turmeric is grown locally; and also in many products such as dairy, beverages, yogurt and many other commonly produced food items. You will also find it in some Asian pickles that contain large chunks of soft turmeric.

Turmeric is not only delectable, it's also great for your skin.

In Chinese and Ayurveda Siddha practices turmeric has been used as medicinal treatment for a variety of ailments and common infections and digestive disorders, and because of its anti-inflammation and anti-bacterial properties, anti-oxidants and UV protecting action, it's widely used in certain parts of the world to accelerate healing in skin conditions such as acne scars, rosacea, psoriasis, skin redness and blotchiness and help to heal wounds.

Turmeric Face Mask that clear and smooth your skin.

This treatment will plump your face and shrink pores and will leave your skin feeling refreshed and rehydrated while adding a natural glow. If you find that your face is stained after use dab cotton in water facial toner and gently wipe.

Add quarter cup milk and one tea spoon of honey, gently heat on a stove or microwave. Add a tea spoon of turmeric and plain yogurt then Mix the ingredients together in a container. Use a pair of gloves to avoid staining of hands from the turmeric. Apply to face for 10 to 20 minutes. Rinse with warm water and pat face dry.

To get benefits of turmeric topically as a moisturizer.

Mix half tea spoon of turmeric, half tea spoon plain yogurt with one table spoon of plain cream solution. Apply to clean face when needed.

Yogurt is made by mixing milk with bacteria (also known as a yogurt starter culture) and letting it culture. During the 1900, a group of scientists started studying and isolating the bacteria that made yogurt. Soon after, they were able to combine selected strains that would culture consistently for commercial produce.

These blends are called direct-set cultures. Yogurt is fermented by a type of culture that produces lactic acid and yogurt when the good active bacteria are added. The culture is of Lactobacillus delbrueckii subsp. bulgaricus and Streptococcus thermophiles a form of healthy bacteria. Other bacteria sweeteners and flavourings are sometimes added.

The milk is heated to around 84 °C (184 °F). The milk then goes through a process that prevents it from curdling. . After heating, the milk is allowed to cool to about 45 °C (113 °F). The bacterial culture is mixed in, and a temperature of 45 °C (113 °F) is maintained for five to ten hours to allow fermentation.

Yogurt is good because it has beneficial bacteria that supports the digestive tract.

Yogurt's popularity in the U S started in the 1950s to 60s when it was introduced as a health food by the scientists Stephen A. Gaymont. By the late 20th century, yogurt had become a common American food item and around the world.

Using Yogurt topically improves the elastin of the skin leaving it bright and clear, while removing dark circles.

Yogurt can help to fight acne.

The yogurt has natural antibacterial and anti-fungal properties. To shrink acne, put some yogurt on cotton buds and rub unto the area that need treatment. Rinse with warm water after 15 to thirty minutes pat face dry.

Helps to slow down aging

The lactic acid in yogurt will help dissolve dead skin cells and tighten wide pores. Mix enough yogurt with one table spoon of organic coconut oil or extra virgin olive oil. Apply to face after thirty minutes rinse with warm water pat face dry.

You can also apply yogurt topically on skin infections such as athlete's foot, ringworm and other breakouts and skin inflammation.

Cow's milk is one of the most popular dairy products around the world but Goat's milk is a much healthier substitute as researches have shown that goat's milk supports good health in many ways. Goat's milk does not cause inflammation and that's why it is easier for people with bowel irritation to drink goat's milk, because the size of the fat molecules in goat's milk is much smaller than those found in cow's milk. This makes goat's milk easier to digest making it good for the health of your stomach.

Even though it's not the most consumed in western societies, goat milk is actually one of the most widely prevalent milk drinks in the rest of the world. Goat milk is rich in calcium and has 33 per cent more mineral than cow's milk. A healthier choice as It's high in calcium and fatty acids but low in cholesterol and absorb nutrients better than cow's milk and may boost your body's immunity against certain types of diseases.

Word has it that goats milk has healing properties similar to olive oil and is acclaimed for keeping high cholesterol in check as it metabolize iron and copper. It also improves memory and is good for the maintenance of the nervous system.

Good for skin. Folklore has it that Cleopatra use to use goat's milk as a beauty treatment for her skin. It is power-packed with proteins and Vitamins A and E that promotes smoother clearer skin.

You can rejuvenate your skin with this simple goat milk bath spa. The lactic acid in milk helps to exfoliate and soften your skin.

This therapeutic bath recipe I learned from my grand-mother when I was a teenager. She lived in the country side in a big farm house and I always had an amazing time when I visited. Surrounded by large farms and forests of trees, and fruit orchards it was easy to get fresh goats milk and fruits from other nearby farmers, and apart from drinking it we used it to pamper and make natural skin products.

It will depend on how much water is in your bath tub, but I add three to five cups of goat milk and some fresh orange peel in a half tub of warm bath water and have a good soak. Goat milk has protein and fats that restore while working its magic on your skin!

 You can also use this other option to treat yourself.

Add two cups of powdered goat milk and one quarter cup of sea salt, soak and gently scrub your skin. The fatty contents and acid in the goat milk work to nourish the skin and the sea salt remove the dead skin.

"Olive oil" is oil obtained from the fruit of olive trees and olive oil has a long history of being used as a home remedy and therapeutic practices dating way back from ancient times, stretching as far back as the Egyptians, Jews and Greeks who use to use it as a moisturizer, cleanser and antibacterial agent; and In ancient Greek, olive oil was used during massage, to prevent sports injuries among competitors, relieve muscle fatigue, and eliminate lactic acid build-up, and commonly used in their cuisine.

During the great Exodus of the tribes of Israel from Egypt it is noted that In Jewish observance, olive oil is the only fuel allowed to be used in the seven-branched Menorah in the Mishkan service and in temples in Jerusalem. It was acquired by using only the first drop from a squeezed olive and was consecrated for use only in the Temple by the priests and was stored in special containers.

Olive oil is also used in the Roman Catholic, Orthodox and Anglican churches, consecration of pulpits and traditionally, in the anointing of coronation.

The olive tree is also native to the Mediterranean when wild olives were collected by Neolithic peoples as early as the 8th millennium BC. In the 1500 BC The hotter the country the stronger the taste of the oil. Extra virgin olive oil is considered the healthiest and purest.

Olive oil is extremely good for you here is why.

People have consuming olive oil for thousands of years and it is now more popular around the world now more than ever as it is known to protect the heart and help to fight cancer and can Help Prevent or Treat Diabetes and help to balance hormones.

Olive oil contains powerful antioxidants known as polyphenols, and extra virgin olive oil is considered an anti-inflammatory food and cardiovascular protector.

For a healthy shiny hair try this olive oil hair mask. Mix two spoons full of olive oil and one spoon full of honey with one egg yolk whip and apply to hair from roots to tip massage in. Put on a steaming cap and shampoo and condition after thirty minutes. If burning or breakout occur while treating skin with turmeric wash immediately.

For rejuvenation of skin

Mix two tea spoonsful of extra virgin olive oil, add a spoonul of plain yogurt and one spoonful of honey and one tea spoon full of brown sugar. Mix until blend apply to face and leave for 10 to 20 minutes. Rinse with warm water. Enjoy beautiful soft silky skin!

Tomato is a watery pulpy fruit of Solanum lycopersicum. The plant belongs to the nightshade family. Tomatoes are powerfully packed with nutrients and antioxidants and are a rich source of vitamins A and C and folic acid, which neutralizes harmful free radicals, and also contain beta-carotene. Tomato fruit is categorized as a berry fruit. The fruit is full of seeds and moisture, called ocular cavities which may vary through cultivation processes. Even-though it's a fruit it is used as a vegetable adding colour and zest to special salads and savoury dishes.

Tomatoes grow in vast quantities and researches have shown that there are lots of different tomato variations. The four best tomatoes grown organically or not are Jet Star, First Lady, New Girl, and Fantastic. Although one one study was conducted this might be a strong indicator that particular types of tomatoes might be of more nutritional value than others.

Eating of tomatoes has long been associated with heart health. Enough consumption of this fruit have been shown to help lower total cholesterol. Tomato is good for the heart because of the folic acid inside the fruit which keep homo-cysteine levels regulated, but for those that suffer from acid influx consumption of the fruit must be eaten in moderation.

After it was introduced to the Middle East by John Barker tomato become a popular part of their cuisine, served fresh in salads and other culinary dishes. Tomatoes were brought to the Caribbean islands by the Spanish during the period of colonization.

Tomato is good for dandruff.

This is really easy, all you have to do is Apply tomato pulp on your scalp for 30 minutes and then wash shampoo and condition hair. The juice from the tomato will also increase the shine texture and colour of the hair.

Tomato rejuvenates skin and helps to remove black heads and impurities while it tightens up the pores.

Mix one spoon full of tomato juice with two drops of orange juice and two drops of lemon juice. Apply to clean face for 15 to 20 minutes, then rinse with Luke warm water pat face dry.

Here is another simple facial.

Chop up one ripe tomato and add two spoons full of lemon and quarter cup oats: blend together in a thick smooth paste. Apply to face for 15 to 20 minutes or as long as you like. Rinse with warm water and pat dry.

About The Author

I am a supporter for green living. I try to promote healthy lifestyle choices whenever I can.